Norbert Salenbauch / Arrigo Cipriani / Volker Kriegel

Al dente

Culinary Delight for the Dental Patient

Recipes, Tips, and Advice

With a Foreword by Frank Celenza

Translation by
Sandro Popelka

Quintessence Publishing Co, Ltd.
London, Berlin, Chicago, Tokyo, Barcelona, Beijing, Istanbul, Milan,
Moscow, New Delhi, Paris, Prague, São Paulo, and Warsaw

British Library Cataloguing in Publication Data
Salenbauch, Norbert
  Al dente : Culinary Delight for the Dental Patient.
  Recipes, Tips, and Advice.
  1. Dental therapeutics - Popular works 2. Cookery
  3. Gastronomy
  I. Title II. Cipriani, Arrigo III. Kriegel, Volker
  617.6

ISBN-13: 9781850971870

© 2009 Quintessence Publishing Co, Ltd

Quintessence Publishing Co, Ltd
Grafton Road
New Malden
Surrey KT3 3AB
United Kingdom
www.quintpub.co.uk

Translation: Dr Sandro Popelka

All rights reserved. This book or any part thereof may not be reproduced, stored in a retrieval system, or transmitted in any form or by any means, electronic, mechanical, photocopying, or otherwise, without prior written permission of the publisher.

Printed in Germany

Contents

Preface 7
Foreword 11
A Note from the Chef 13
General Advice 15
The First Sign of Trouble 21
Coping with Pain Safely 25
Tooth Sensitivity 34
Facing the Neglect of Your Teeth 41
Preparing for Your Restorative Treatment .. 45
Simple Tooth Extraction 57
Surgical Tooth Extraction 61
Antibiotics 73
Provisional Teeth 77
Gum Surgery 83
The Joy of Dental Implants 89
Your New Teeth 99
Closing Remarks 104

Preface

The process of eating begins the moment that food passes through the tactile barrier of your lips. Your sense of taste is enhanced by what you see and smell before your taste organs complete this pleasurable experience. It is the coordinated orchestration by your tongue, palate, and teeth that makes food so flavorful and eating so enjoyable.

We appreciate our ability to enjoy eating most when it is disabled. Only then is the value of a healthy mouth fully realized. For whatever reason, if you are in such discomfort or pain that you have to focus on carefully handling certain foods with your tongue so that they don't touch your gums and parts of your teeth, it is difficult to enjoy eating. A tasteful meal requires a functional, pain-free chewing apparatus and functional taste organs. Culinary delights are able to spread their aroma only when they are freely chewed by teeth and then pressed by the taste buds on the tongue and palate. The obstruction of chewing and taste sensation by pain or dental appliances compromises the enjoyment of the eating experience.

If you wear a denture, your ability to taste is blocked by acrylic resin or metal in the areas of taste sensation. Maybe you have gotten used to the dullness of flavor; perhaps you do not consider yourself a connoisseur. Or, maybe, your dentist has not introduced you to recent developments in dentistry. Dental implants have made taste-killing dentures a relic of another era. You may not be able to exert the biting force necessary to enjoy food. Or your teeth and gums start hurting every time you eat warm or cold foods and sweet or sour foods.

Older people, especially, may have difficulty sensing taste fully. The expression "eating is sex at a later age" may be an exaggeration, but it still brings the point across: Eating is an enjoyable experience that means more than just food intake. To be able to savor tasteful meals as an older person would be a significant improvement in quality of life.

Most of us look at food as more than just fuel—we look forward to meals, we have cravings that tempt us throughout the day, we expel a pleasurable sigh when we take that first delicious bite after the hours of fasting between meals. And we are disappointed if our expectations of taste are dashed for whatever reason. There are those who just want to eat what is easy and fast. A diet revolving around TV dinners, fast food, packaged snacks, and microwaved meals has become routine for a lot of people. At the same time, the appreciation of gourmet food is just as prevalent. Wherever you look, there are gourmet restaurants and food stores, television cooking programs, and glossy cooking magazines that celebrate notable chefs, their glorious creations, and the art of eating well. The average household is trying out dishes that high-end chefs are demonstrating. You, too, can prepare haute cuisine without the hefty price tag. Many people have discovered the art of cooking as an enjoyable part of their everyday life. It is unfortunate that people with an improperly functioning chewing apparatus feel that they have to eat bland mush, when they could be enjoying food as much as they had before.

I have heard patients say, "At least I can lose some weight." This is certainly not the time to give up on nutritional values, though. A weakened, nutritionally deprived patient responds far worse to treatment and healing than a well-nourished, happy person; comprehensive dental treatment can take months or even years. Therefore, it is very important for patients to keep their strength and spirits up by pampering themselves with tantalizing cuisine! The inspiration for this book comes from an older couple who are patients of mine. Both partners are passionate hunters and they love good food. As gourmet food lovers, they do not want to be deprived of this source of enjoyment. It is interesting how well, and with joy, this couple dines on a regular basis. With an endless variety of exquisite recipes, it is possible to continue enjoying good food while enduring extensive dental treatment with the accompanying oral sensitivity, provisional teeth, and soreness.

So, I hope that this "survival guide for patients undergoing dental treatment" inspires you to stock your cupboards in preparation for your treatment and to make eating an enjoyable part of each day. Cheers!

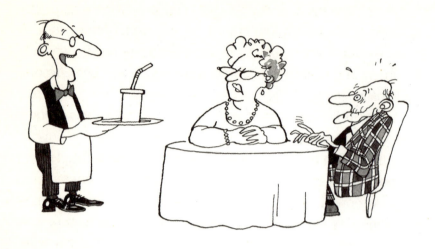

Foreword

I consider it an honor and a privilege to write this foreword for Dr Salenbauch's "cook book," *Al dente*.

I have considered writing such a book many times, since I pride myself as a gourmet cook. Certainly, it is a natural thing for a prosthodontist to have a serious interest in the culinary arts. This is not only for the dentition and its function but, more importantly, because of the artistic and inventive elements common to both fields.

No book on the culinary arts would be complete without an analysis of the world's great cuisines. We can divide this topic into two categories: provincial cuisines and haute cuisine. For the most part, provincial cuisines occupy the most attention, some more prominently than others. Every provincial cuisine shows influences from the cultures that have overrun them through history. In my view, there are three great provincial cuisines: Chinese, French, and Italian. Recently, American cuisine has come into the picture, but all the rest make major contributions that fall somewhat short on their own. The melding of provincial cuisines is called *fusion*. Simply stated, provincial cuisines are dependent on local food availability and supply and undergo modifications and refinements over the years. This is home-style cooking, which is at once individual, innovative, and most enjoyable because of its simplicity and freshness.

The other cuisine is French haute cuisine, which set the standard for scientific classification and artistic involvement.

In this cuisine, consistency and precision are paramount. The techniques and standards should be the same regardless of the location. Yet recently, even this cuisine is changing, and artistic innovations are enhancing the basic foundations established by the originators such as Marie-Antoine Carême and Georges Auguste Escoffier, among others.* This new cuisine is an advancement over the old standards but always at a high level. This is as it should be and can only spur interest and inventiveness, which is how all art forms have evolved.

Caterina de Medici brought the Florentine cuisine to France in 1533 when she married the future King Henry II. This is why Italian cuisine has been called *la cucina madre*—a reminder that it was the mother of the developing French art form.

So, with all of this history that contributed greatly to masticatory efficiency, occlusal precision, and out-and-out enjoyment, it is a great pleasure and certainly an honor to be a part of this wonderful undertaking.

Frank Celenza, DDS, PC

They set the rules and classified all categories in great detail. They organized the kitchen staff into various departments such as saucier, sous-chef, etc.

A Note from the Chef

When I was 20, a dentist from Venice took me aside and, nodding his head to reinforce his words, said to me, "Dear Arrigo, I can tell you that you will not die with your teeth."

Lots of time has gone by since then. The old doctor met his end a few years ago, hopefully with all his teeth still intact. I am now 76, and I am sorry that I cannot tell him to his face that, so far, he has been wrong. With the exception of my wisdom teeth, all my teeth are still in my mouth, doing their job, and they give no sign of giving up.

Whether this is due to the fact that I eat most of my meals at Harry's Bar or to some other unknown reason, I cannot say. Dr Salenbauch seems certain that my food has something to do with it. Let him think so.

I hope you will enjoy some of these recipes that have been selected to make your life happier and to reassure you as you eat following dental treatment.

Best wishes,
Arrigo Cipriani

General Advice

At one time it was recommended to be especially careful right after the placement of new dental restorations. Today this is not necessary, because once the patient leaves the dental chair, modern fillings have fully hardened. An exception is the very rarely used amalgam fillings. Nevertheless, some basic rules need to be followed throughout the healing process to avoid any complications. By adhering to the following recommendations, your eating habits during the treatment and recovery phases should not interfere with your enjoyment or healing.

Two important preliminary precautions bear mentioning before any other: First, never eat while your mouth is numb! You can injure yourself badly by biting yourself without the warning of pain. Second, call your dentist immediately if any critical complications arise at any time.

Food consistency

Avoid hard foods. When you are craving that crusty baguette or a jagged piece of almond brittle, imagine the pain and potential damage to your freshly healing wounds that biting into and chewing such foods will cause. Other items that should be avoided include food containing small hard pieces of seasonings or other bits, such as whole wheat kernels, peppercorns, and seeds. Even in soft cakes and jams, seeds and other hard particles can get lodged into the wound and hinder the healing process. The use of a liquid rinse after eating can be beneficial. It does not always have to be water—wine can serve the purpose! We will address this topic later.

Temperature triggers

When the nerves beneath the teeth are stimulated by hot or cold foods and beverages, pain may result, even in people with healthy mouths. This jarring pain is caused by stimulation of the *tooth cervix*, or the area where the enamel meets the root. The tooth cervix is exposed when the gum line recedes, due to age or other factors. The gum line can be harmed by orthodontic braces and retainers or other appliances, as well as by improper brushing techniques. It is especially irritating when a necessary dental procedure leads to some recession at the gum line. Nevertheless, sensitivity at the tooth cervix can be easily treated in most cases. In some cases, a surgical procedure may be necessary to cover the exposed areas with healthy gum tissue. Meanwhile, there is a simple solution: Stay away from foods that are too hot or too cold!

Chemical triggers

Very sweet, sour, salty, and spicy foods can irritate sensitive areas and affect the healing process. For the defective or healing oral cavity, liquids and solids whose chemical makeup closely resembles the chemical contents of blood are the most comfortable to consume. In general, blood can be described as a lightly salted solution of water. Any deviation from this chemical makeup can cause pain, depending on the stage of the illness and healing. A fruit smoothie, considered a healthy cocktail under normal circumstances, is most definitely too sour in this situation. And like fruits and fruit juices, vegetables and vegetable juices are also too caustic.

Milk products should also be avoided. This precaution is especially important during the first 3 days following the intervention. Why? There is a large amount of bacteria in the oral cavity that are normally very useful and even essential to keep a healthy oral environment. Some of these bacteria break down milk products, causing them to rot in the mouth. This process is detrimental to wound healing. Therefore during the first 3 days after surgery, keep away from milk, yogurt, cream, cream cheese, and milk shakes!

Healing solution

If your wounds encounter any of the above triggers, there is a remedy. Immediately after eating, rinse your mouth out with mildly warm saltwater to loosen food particles and to neutralize the oral chemistry. Commercial mouthrinses should be avoided, especially during the first 3 days following a dental procedure, as they contain additional ingredients that may interfere with the healing process. Simple, warm saltwater is highly recommended as a healing mouthrinse.

Minestrone

Vegetable Soup

Minestrone is a mellow vegetable soup, and its composition depends on using the best vegetables available. This healthful and inexpensive minestrone is all vegetables. For a true vegetarian soup, use water instead of chicken stock. This minestrone recipe produces a light, thin consistency. The composite taste is a blend of all the elements, but each vegetable retains its flavor.

Serves 6 as a first course
2 tablespoons olive oil
2 tablespoons unsalted butter
1 medium onion, diced
1 large celery rib, cut into ¼-inch dice
2 leeks, white part only, thoroughly washed and thinly sliced
1 large tomato, cored and cut into ¼-inch dice
2 small zucchini, cut into ¼-inch dice
a small wedge of green or Savoy cabbage coarsely chopped
1 medium potato, peeled and cut into ¼-inch dice
1 medium carrot, peeled and cut into ¼-inch dice
6 asparagus spears, cut into ¼-inch slices
1 bay leaf
salt
freshly ground pepper
2 quarts boiling water or chicken stock
⅓ cup tomato sauce
freshly grated Parmesan cheese

Heat the olive oil in a soup pot over medium heat, and melt 1 tablespoon of the butter in it. Add the onion, and sauté over medium-low heat, stirring frequently, until it is well browned—10 to 15 minutes. Add the remaining vegetables, the bay leaf, and a little salt and pepper. Continue to cook, stirring the vegetables frequently with a wooden spoon, for 15 minutes. Add the water or stock and the tomato sauce. Bring the soup to a boil, reduce the heat, and simmer, partially covered, for 15 minutes. Remove the bay leaf, and thin the soup with a little boiling water if it is too thick. Stir in the remaining tablespoon of butter, taste the soup, and adjust the seasoning. Serve very hot and pass a bowl of grated Parmesan cheese.

Wine notes
Italian: Tocai—Livio Felluga
American: Chardonnay—Callaway

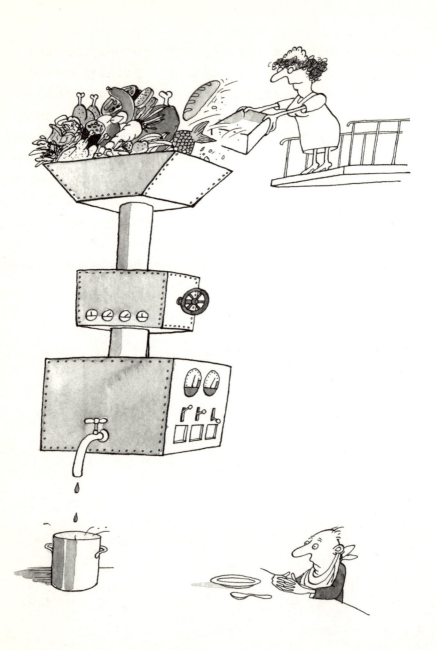

The First Sign of Trouble

You can't ignore a problem away. When that on-again/off-again pain finally becomes unbearable during dinner one day, your body, which had been nagging up until that point, is now screaming for help. Or when you bite with weakened teeth and they finally fracture, it is really no surprise, is it? Now you regret not taking your dentist's advice to replace your aged restorations with a stronger, more solid material. By the way, if a chip of filling or tooth is mixed in with your food and you can't stop the process of swallowing, you need not worry, because it will be excreted naturally.

If the first sign of distressful pain is triggered by dessert, and you are at a formal dinner, just pick up your glass of water instead of another spoonful of mousse. Rinse your mouth—discreetly—to dilute the concentration of this chemical trigger and to remove the irritating substance. You can overcome these uncomfortable situations without drawing attention to yourself, but you may have to excuse yourself and go to the bathroom if pieces of food are severely lodged. Careful cleaning with a toothbrush or dental floss can relieve the pain. Use only a minimal amount of toothpaste, though, if any. Even if the pain subsides, it is time to visit your dentist! The pain you have been feeling now and then is a sign that something is wrong. Procrastination will only make the problem bigger. Instead of a simple filling, a complicated root canal may be necessary by the time you seek help. After making an appointment, you can prepare for your visit through good oral hygiene, avoidance of temperature and chemical triggers, and keeping to a soothing diet.

Ravioli di Magro alla Salvia

Spinach and Cheese Ravioli with Sage

There are countless ways to prepare ravioli, but one of the best is this very simple dish from a restaurant in the little town of Valeggio sul Mincio near Lake Garda. Make this dish only if you can get fresh sage.

Serves 6 as a first course or 4 as a main course
1 tablespoon salt
1 recipe ravioli with spinach and cheese filling
4 tablespoons unsalted butter
18 fresh sage leaves
6 tablespoons freshly grated Parmesan cheese, plus extra to pass at the table

Bring a large pot of water to a boil and add the salt. Drop in the ravioli and cook them for 6 to 8 minutes—the ravioli should not be al dente; they should be quite tender. Drain them well in a colander. While the ravioli are cooking, chop 12 of the sage leaves. Melt 3 tablespoons of the butter in a large skillet and sauté the chopped sage over medium-high heat until the foam starts to subside. Remove the skillet with half the Parmesan. Toss well and transfer the mixture to a heated serving platter. To the same skillet, add the remaining tablespoon of butter and the 6 whole sage leaves and cook over high heat for 30 seconds. Sprinkle the rest of the Parmesan on the ravioli, pour on the butter and sage mixture, and serve immediately. Pass around a small bowl of grated Parmesan cheese.

For the ravioli:

1 egg
1 recipe of dough for egg pasta, kneaded and rolled into strips
2 cups filling

Lay a strip of pasta dough on a lightly floured surface. Trim off any uneven ends of the dough and cut it in half to make 2 strips approximately 4½ by 12 inches each. Using a pastry brush, paint the entire surface of one of the strips with beaten egg. Place very small mounds of filling—no more than a rounded ½ teaspoon each—on the dough. Make 2 rows of mounds approximately 1 inch apart and leave at least ½ inch of pasta around all the edges. Cover this with the second half of the strip. Press the dough very firmly around all the edges and between the mounds of filling to seal the ravioli. Using the pastry wheel or ravioli cutter, cut all around the outside edge of the filled strip to seal it; then cut the strip into 2-inch squares and place them on a lightly floured surface. Repeat with the remaining dough and filling.

If you are not going to cook the ravioli right away, place them in one layer on well-floured baking sheets, cover with plastic wrap, and refrigerate. To freeze ravioli, place the baking sheet in the freezer until the ravioli are frozen. Put the frozen ravioli in plastic bags and seal tightly.

For the filling:
Makes about 2½ cups
½ 10-oz package frozen chopped spinach, thawed and squeezed dry
½ cup whole-milk ricotta
½ cup grated Swiss cheese
¼ pound whole-milk mozzarella, diced
¼ cup freshly grated Parmesan cheese
1 teaspoon salt
freshly ground pepper
⅛ teaspoon cayenne pepper
2 egg yolks

Place the spinach, ricotta, Swiss cheese, mozzarella, and Parmesan in a food processor fitted with a steel blade, and process it until just combined. Scrape the mixture into a bowl and blend in the salt, pepper, cayenne pepper, and egg yolks. Taste and adjust the seasoning. Cover the bowl with plastic wrap and refrigerate until you are ready to use it.

Wine notes
Italian: Greco di Tufo—Mastroberardino
American: Sauvignon Blanc—BV

Coping with Pain Safely

Pain is a protective warning against physical and mental damage to our body. It is perceived differently by each person no matter how large or small the cause is. Some people are more sensitive to pain than others. The perception of pain can depend on your mental as well as physical status.

Pain can drive us insane. The opposite can be true as well—mental suffering can cause pain of the jawbone and the masticatory system. The pain finally subsides, though, when the causative stress diminishes. On the contrary, we know of the fakir who sits on a bed of nails and, through mental control and meditation, does not feel pain. This example supports the idea that pain is not an objective measure but rather a subjective feeling, influenced by individual factors. Therefore, the simplified idea of tooth pain traveling through the nerve pathway to the brain and causing an unbearable pain is not realistic. Pain operates through a complex nervous system that can trigger a variety of painful sensations. A dentist may not understand what an unbearable toothache feels like, since dentists are highly motivated to perform good oral hygiene and therefore often do not experience dental pain. However, we do sympathize with you in your state of severe pain and recognize the outward appearance of suffering: the sweating forehead, ashen skin, and tense facial expressions. The relief of pain is our immediate goal.

Once you are seated in the dental chair, the relief of acute pain is technically no problem. The modern anesthetics are very successful in achieving rapid numbness. Nevertheless,

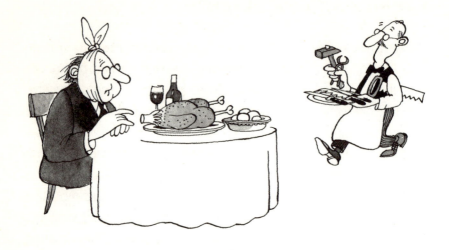

before the dental visit you probably feel rather helpless. The pain medication from your medicine cabinet and the over-the-counter remedies have not provided the expected relief, especially not for the long term. You have probably avoided eating, and as a result the pain medications have upset your stomach. At this point, you are relieved to be sitting in the dental chair. You never thought you'd be so happy to see the dentist—but you have recognized that you really need professional help and understanding to get you through this oral crisis.

The numerous household remedies and self-cure medications that are in use portray how painful a toothache can be. Even the simplest of practical recommendations can provide some relief and change mood.

There are many self-help alternatives that my patients have told me about through the years. For example, a patient handed me a book in which cherry schnapps is recommended for a toothache. The directions call for a combination of 34 ounces of cherry brandy; a tablespoon of refined salt, sea salt, and iodized salt (with a ratio of 1:3); and some lukewarm water for use in the oral cavity. The patient did not say whether the solution should be used as a rinse or taken internally, but she mentioned that the solution could also be massaged into the forehead for pain relief. Furthermore, she told me about another old household remedy—placing clove directly onto the affected tooth—to promote healing. The sedating power of alcohol on nerves and the brain is of course widely recognized.

The temperature of any remedy has to be carefully evaluated. Not all kinds of toothaches can be relieved through heat. In general, cooling treatments bring relief to inflamed tooth and gum tissues. Temperature affects the rate of blood circulation and nerve transmission. Everybody knows that ice-cold hands lose their feeling and that warm body parts are far more sensitive. Inflamed tissue has increased temperature and blood circulation compared with normal tissue; therefore, cold temperatures will decrease the circulation and the nerve transmission rate and lower the pressure in the tissue.

The soft tissue inside an aching tooth cannot expand, as inflamed tissue normally does, and therefore it exerts pressure inside the hollow space within the tooth. This pressure can be so strong that the tooth slightly bulges out of its socket. Do not snap you teeth together in this instance! An ice pack (rather than pain medication) will decrease the pressure and therefore reduce the pain.

Heat treatment is helpful if the jaw joint, muscles, or nerves (neuralgia) are involved.

By asking you what helps alleviate the pain best—cold or heat—your dentist will be better able to determine the source of the pain. If coldness brings relief, it is likely that the cause of the pain is located in or on the tooth. If heat brings relief, the surrounding tissue, muscles, or nerves are likely involved.

Persistent pain can disrupt our emotional and cognitive well-being, especially when we are avoiding food on top of everything else. Well-being depends partly on a contented stomach, after all! Besides, good, nourishing food can help us refocus and cope better with pain. After an emergency visit to the dentist, food intake is not possible for a few hours, or at least until the anesthetic wears off. But regular food intake before and after is crucial for successful treatment and recovery. The digestive system, and therefore nutritional status, is at risk when only pain medication and water are consumed over a period of time, without any food.

Risotto alla Primavera

Risotto with Vegetables Primavera

This dish calls for about half of the vegetables primavera (see below) recipe. It is suggested that you cook the whole amount and freeze half. That way you can make Risotto alla Primavera on the spur of the moment.

Serves 6 as a first course
1 recipe risotto parmigiano (see below)
3 cups cooked vegetables primavera (see below)
freshly grated Parmesan cheese

Prepare risotto parmigiano as directed in the basic recipe, adding the cooked vegetables halfway through the cooking of the rice, or after about 10 minutes. Serve immediately, passing around a small bowl of grated Parmesan cheese.

For the risotto parmigiano:

Serves 6 as a first course
5 to 6 cups chicken stock, preferably homemade
1 tablespoon olive oil
1 small onion, minced
1½ cups short-grain Italian rice, preferably Vialone or Carnaroli
3 tablespoons unsalted butter at room temperature
⅔ cup freshly grated Parmesan cheese, plus extra to pass at the table

salt
freshly ground pepper

Bring the stock to a simmer in a saucepan and keep it at a bare simmer.

Heat the olive oil in a heavy-bottomed 3-quart saucepan and cook the onion over medium heat, stirring until the onion is golden but not brown, about 3 to 5 minutes. Add the rice and stir with a wooden spoon to coat the rice well with the oil and onion. Turn the heat to medium high, add about ½ cup of the simmering stock, and keep the mixture boiling, stirring constantly. As soon as the stock has been absorbed, add another ½ cup of stock and stir until it is absorbed. You may have to adjust the heat from time to time; the risotto has to keep boiling, but it must not stick to the pot. If it does stick, put the pot on a Flame Tamer. Continue adding stock, about ½ cup at a time, stirring constantly and waiting until each portion is absorbed before adding the next, until the rice is creamy and tender on the outside, with each grain still distinct and firm.

This process will take at least 15 minutes, depending on your pot and your stove. If the rice is still a bit hard in the middle after you have used all but a few tablespoons of the stock, add boiling water ¼ cup at a time, stirring it in as you did the stock, until each grain of rice is tender but still has the slightest bit of firmness and the mixture is creamy.

Remove the pan from the heat and vigorously stir in the butter and the Parmesan. This stirring will make the risotto even creamier. Taste and season with salt and pepper. While continuing to stir vigorously, add the few remaining tablespoons of hot stock (or boiling water if you've used all the stock) to make the consistency softer and softer. Taste carefully for seasoning and serve immediately, passing a small bowl of grated Parmesan cheese.

For the vegetables primavera:

Makes about 7 cups

¼ cup olive oil
1 garlic clove, crushed
2 cups thinly sliced shiitake mushroom caps
6 baby artichokes or 1 large artichoke, trimmed and sliced
2 tablespoons finely chopped onion
4 small zucchini, cut into ¼-inch dice
12 asparagus spears, trimmed and cut into ½-inch slices
½ red bell pepper, cut into ¼-inch dice
2 medium plum tomatoes, cut into ¼-inch dice
1 medium leek, white part only, thoroughly washed and cut into ¼-inch dice
salt
freshly ground pepper

Heat the oil in a large skillet over medium heat. Add the garlic, cook it for 30 seconds to flavor the oil, and then discard it. Add the mushrooms and cook for 5 or 6 minutes, until they are softened and the liquid has evaporated. Add the artichokes and cook until tender—8 to 10 minutes. Add the onion and cook for another 2 minutes.

Add the zucchini, asparagus, bell pepper, tomatoes, and leek; raise the heat and cook for another 10 minutes, stirring frequently until the vegetables are just cooked. Season the vegetables with salt and pepper.

For the artichokes:

For the recipes in this book, use either large artichokes or baby ones. You will use only the hearts of the large artichokes. The inner leaves of the baby artichokes are tender enough to leave attached to the hearts, and they have no chokes.

1 large artichoke heart, sliced, makes ½ cup
4 or 5 baby artichokes, trimmed and sliced, makes ½ cup

Have ready a large bowl half-filled with cold water and the juice of half a large lemon.

To prepare large artichokes: Cut off the stem even with the base of the artichoke. Bend the outer leaves back until they snap off close to the base. Repeat with layers of the leaves until you reach the tender, pale innermost layers of leaves. Slice off the top of the artichoke, leaving about an inch attached to the heart. Cut the artichoke in half lengthwise. Using a sharp knife point, cut out the choke and remove the sharp little leaves. Drop the artichoke into the bowl of acidulated water and repeat the process with the remaining artichokes. Remove the artichoke halves from the water one at a time, trim all remaining bits of green leaves from the outer edge, and cut the heart lengthwise into thin slices. Return the slices to the bowl of water and repeat the process until all of the artichoke hearts have been sliced.

Drain the sliced artichokes, spread them out on paper towels, and pat dry. They are now ready to use.

To prepare baby artichokes: Cut off the stem even with the base of the artichoke. Bend back the outer leaves until they snap off close to the base. Repeat until all the green leaves are gone, leaving the tender yellow-green inner leaves attached to the bottom. Slice off the top of the artichoke, leaving about 1½ inches, and put it in the bowl of acidulated water. Repeat the process with the remaining artichokes.

Remove the artichokes from the water one at a time and cut them in half lengthwise. As you will see, baby artichokes have no chokes. Cut each half lengthwise into 3 or 4 wedges and return the wedges to the bowl of water. When all the artichokes have been sliced, drain them, spread them out on paper towels, and pat dry. They are now ready to use.

Wine notes

Italian: Chardonnay—Maculan
American: Chardonnay—Zaca Mesa

Tooth Sensitivity

The sensitive cervical areas, where the enamel meets the gum, react to various adverse stimulants. If you have sensitivity in these areas, you may relate to the following story.

It was late winter, and a seemingly endless bout of influenza kept me in bed. I felt obligated to make a profound change in my way of living so that I would perhaps heal more quickly and be better equipped to fight off a later attack. With a weakened body driven by high motivation, I managed to get to the grocery store, where I bought loads of fruit, especially citrus fruits. The flu bug proved itself to be a persistent one, but I fought bravely by eating as many fruits as I could.

During those weeks I noticed that my teeth were not functioning properly. It was painful to chew and to brush my teeth. I figured the problem was due to my weakened condition, because my oral hygiene practices were excellent. After a few weeks of citrus therapy, the flu was almost cured, but the tooth pain was still there. I was scared to brush my teeth and to drink anything cold. Even the thought of drinking a nice cold beer was dampened by negative expectations.

When I fully recovered from the flu, I continued to celebrate my newfound dedication to live a healthier life (meaning: enough sleep, alcohol in moderation, no nicotine, athletic activity, and a healthy diet), and I went on a skiing trip. One morning while downhill skiing, I was laughing out of happiness, with my mouth open, and a rush of cold air into my mouth caused a sudden toothache that overcame me! The cruel blow confused and depressed me. Here I was, happy and healthy—so why was I in pain? And how ironic was it that my happy laughter triggered it!

At that time I was at the start of of my professional career, and I could not understand how a healthy diet could permanently damage the hard tissue of the tooth. Today when I hear health-conscious patients proudly proclaim that they start each day with fruits and juices but complain about suffering pain at the tooth cervix, I can explain the connection.

If you have marble countertops in your kitchen, you know how dangerous lime juice is to the surfaces. Compare a healthy tooth surface with your marble countertop. If a drop of acid drips onto it without being diluted and removed immediately, the shine will

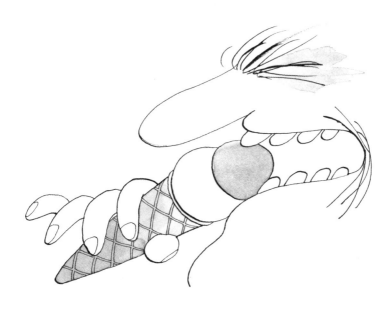

vanish. If you let the acid sit or if you remove it with pressure through rubbing, a concavity will be created. That is exactly what happens when acids from food react with the tooth surface. The increased consumption of fruits such as lemon, pineapple, grapefruit, and oranges can harm the protective layer of enamel at the tooth cervix and therefore expose the underlying dentin, and its nerve canals.

Your dentist needs to know about your daily eating habits to determine, for example, whether acidic foods are routinely consumed before the episodes of painful brushing.

The electrifying pain with triggering stimuli will subside if you routinely rinse your mouth with warm saltwater after eating acidic foods to neutralize the tooth surfaces. In case you do not have a neutralizing rinse handy (such as when dining in a restaurant, taking off in a rush after a meal at a friend's house, or leaving a family get-together), it is recommended to chew sugar-free gum. When you chew gum, excess saliva is produced, which will neutralize the effect of the acid, through its buffering capacity. Therefore it makes sense to always have a pack of sugar-free gum handy—in places where gum chewing is acceptable, of course. The intimate atmosphere of your car is perfectly suited for such occasions. After breakfast on the way to work, after lunch on the way back to work, or after dining in a restaurant on the way home—sugar-free gum should always be accessible.

Cape Sante al Curry e Tagliolini

Scallops with Curry Sauce and Green Tagliolini

Serves 6 as a main course
2 pounds of bay scallops
salt
freshly ground pepper
flour for dredging
3 tablespoons olive oil
2 tablespoons brandy
curry sauce, made with fish stock (see below)
½ cup heavy cream

Rinse the scallops and dry them well. Then season them with salt and pepper, dredge them in flour, and shake them in a sieve to remove excess flour. Heat the oil in a large skillet over high heat. Add the scallops, in batches if necessary, and cook them, tossing constantly, until they are lightly browned—4 to 7 minutes. Pour off the oil, add the brandy, warm it, and carefully ignite it. Swirl the skillet until the flames die out.

Add the curry sauce and the cream to the pan and cook, stirring, until the sauce and scallops are hot.

For the curry sauce:
Makes about 3 cups
¼ cup olive oil
1 small onion, chopped

2 leeks, white part only, thoroughly washed and thinly sliced
1 celery rib, chopped
1 Golden Delicious apple, peeled, cored, and thinly sliced
3 tablespoons brandy
salt
freshly ground pepper
2 to 3 teaspoons curry powder, to taste
¼ cup flour
3 cups boiling fish stock
½ cup heavy cream

Heat the oil in a large skillet over medium heat. Add the onion, leeks, and celery and cook for 6 or 7 minutes, until they are wilted. Add the apple and cook the mixture, stirring from time to time, for about 30 minutes, until everything is soft. Pour on the brandy, warm it, and carefully ignite it. Swirl the skillet until the flames die out.

Add some salt and pepper, the curry powder, and the flour, stir well, and cook for 2 or 3 minutes. Whisk in the hot stock and cook the sauce, continuing to whisk, until it thickens. Lower the heat and let the sauce simmer gently, uncovered, for 20 to 30 minutes, stirring frequently.

Strain the sauce into a saucepan. It should be a thin cream sauce with a delicate curry flavor. Adjust the seasoning with salt, pepper, and curry powder. If it is too thick, stir in a little more stock. Bring the cream to a boil in a small saucepan and add it to the sauce. Season the sauce to taste with salt and pepper and let it simmer gently for another 10 minutes.

Curry sauce will keep for 3 or 4 days in the refrigerator and also freezes well.

For ¾ pound green pasta:
¼ cup unbleached white flour
¼ cup durum wheat flour
½ cup fresh or frozen spinach, cooked, drained, squeezed (until very dry), and chopped
1 large egg

Pour the 2 flours into the bowl of a food processor fitted with a steel blade. Turn on the motor. Add the spinach and flour and process until it is evenly distributed. Then add the egg and process for another minute or so. The mixture will look grainy and will stick together when pressed between the fingers.

Pour the mixture into a bowl and press it down to make a solid mass. Gather it up and knead it by hand for a minute or 2. Form a cylinder of dough and cut it into 6 equal pieces. Put the dough in a plastic bag and let it rest for 30 minutes. Have ready several sheets—at least 2 feet long—of lightly floured wax paper. Set the smooth rollers of a pasta machine as far apart as possible, at the highest or lowest number, depending on your machine. Put a little pile of flour on the work surface. Take a piece of dough out of the bag, knead it by hand for a minute or so, and flatten it into a rough rectangle. Dip the dough into the flour and knead in a little extra flour if it is at all sticky. Feed the dough through the roller 9 or 10 times to knead it very thoroughly, folding it in half each time and dusting it lightly with flour if it's sticky.

When the dough has been well kneaded and feels firm and satiny, turn the dial up or down one notch and feed it through the rollers without folding. If the dough is at all sticky, dust it very lightly with flour. Continue to feed the dough through the rollers without folding, turning the dial one notch higher or lower each time, until you reach the next-to-last setting. The dough will be a smooth, long sheet, 4 or 5 inches wide and about 2 feet long. Lay the finished strip on the floured wax paper while you knead and roll the remaining pasta dough. Cover the sheets of dough with wax paper to keep them from drying out.

To make tagliolini: Feed the sheets of dough through the cutting roller to make tagliolini (narrow). Lay the pasta over racks or on lightly floured wax paper to dry slightly before cooking, or let it dry completely and store it in an airtight container or a paper bag.

Cook ¾ pound of green tagliolini. Toss it with 2 tablespoons of unsalted butter and put it on a heated platter. Pour the curried scallops over the pasta and serve immediately.

Wine notes
Italian: Pinot Bianco—Tiefenbrunner
American: Chardonnay—Mazzocco

Facing the Neglect of Your Teeth

It is surprising how our teeth are able to perform for decades despite periods of neglect in caring for them. We expect a lot from our teeth—to help us eat, speak, and smile beautifully at all times. But of course even the most healthy teeth will get sick if not cared for.

Patients across the age spectrum meet with their own age-related dental concerns—and obstacles. As children, our parents remind us to brush our teeth every morning and night and make sure we go to the dentist regularly. This oversight is why most of our teeth survive childhood without illness. Our parents may even take us to get braces to fulfill our ideal picture of how teeth should appear, and encourage an optimal start to the adult world.

In college some of the hygiene rituals instilled by our parents are sacrificed because of stress or change in lifestyle, including regular cleanings and checkups at the dentist as well as consistent use of floss. Initially, these changes may not seem to make a difference. Maybe you have to have a quick filling, and later the wisdom teeth start to make their presence known. A busy student may ignore a toothache too long because there is never a convenient time to go to the dentist. Then, while on vacation in Greece, toothache requires a trip to the local dentist, who can only prescribe high doses of antibiotics. If after the vacation the pain and swelling are gone, the student may not follow up with treatment until the toothache starts up again, maybe during exam week. Incredible timing! If the dentist recommends a root canal and the student again does not have time, the dentist may only be able to treat the problem with a temporary filling. Continued neglect could lead to tooth fracture and necessary surgical extraction.

"Not enough time" remains a factor as the student moves into the working world, and wishful thinking is introduced in the young adult's (lack of) health consciousness. Occasional bleeding of the gums, especially after brushing, might not be enough to convince a young adult that dental care is important at all ages. Some will respond to the bleeding by stepping up their oral care. But most will reduce brushing and flossing, hoping that the gums will heal and unknowingly encouraging a number of dental problems that, if left unchecked, will require extensive treatment.

The years of on-and-off neglect and poor oral hygiene habits begin to catch up with us between the ages of 30 and 45. Disease or other complications may manifest at this point or down the road a bit. The persistent bleeding of the gums is a sign of inflammation, rather than a sign of injury, and is caused by a buildup of plaque and bacteria between the teeth. Other problems, such as defective teeth, old fillings, and partially impacted wisdom teeth are also among the findings starting at the age of 30. A thorough examination may also reveal a deep pocket between some of the teeth. In those areas, the natural bond between gum and tooth has loosened. When the body is no longer able to fight the massive amounts of bacterial poisoning caused by the accumulated plaque, the tissue between the teeth cannot be saved. A patient who rinses the mouth with warm water right after each meal while the food particles are still loose will neutralize acidic

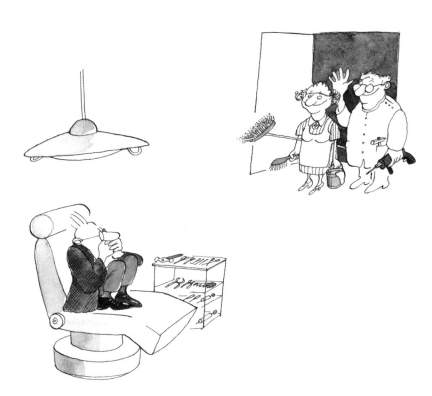

food that can harm the teeth. However, rinsing can remove loose food particles only, and any remaining particles will promote plaque buildup from bacteria. After 24 hours the bacteria develop a toxin, which is able to permanently damage the gum and the supporting tissue. Most people have an effective immune system that is able to fight and neutralize such toxins. As the body defenses begin to weaken in patients after the age of 30, it becomes paramount that patients clean their teeth at least once every 24 hours to remove all plaque and particles, even between teeth.

The best care that dentists can give to their patients is to educate them about preventive care. You may think that all dentists are concerned with prevention, but the hands-on education of dentists since the beginning of the profession has had to focus on the repair of broken teeth. However, more and more dentists today understand the importance of prevention.

Preparing for Your Restorative Treatment

No matter your situation, you should pay extra attention to your oral hygiene to prevent further damage to your teeth and gums. You need to brush and floss daily. Also remember, it is helpful to remove loose particles of food by rinsing your mouth immediately after eating.

The dentist will show you with a mirror how to use floss effectively without hurting the gums and recommend that you practice the technique. Before any restorative dental treatment, the dentist will advise that the teeth be professionally cleaned by a hygienist. Not only will this give you another chance to learn and practice the proper techniques of brushing and flossing, it will bring your teeth and gums into the best possible repair to face any reconstruction.

No matter how attentive you are in your home dental care, bacterial plaque persists, especially in hard-to-reach areas. Even after you have completed treatment, it is important to supplement your home dental care with a professional cleaning on a regular basis. Patients who practice regular oral hygiene and undergo regular professional cleanings have a good chance of retaining their teeth, implants, and restorations for the rest of their life.

The process of removing the plaque increases the sensitivity temporarily in some areas, especially at the cervix where tooth and gum meet, and in areas below the gum line where the plaque has dissolved the protective bond between gum and

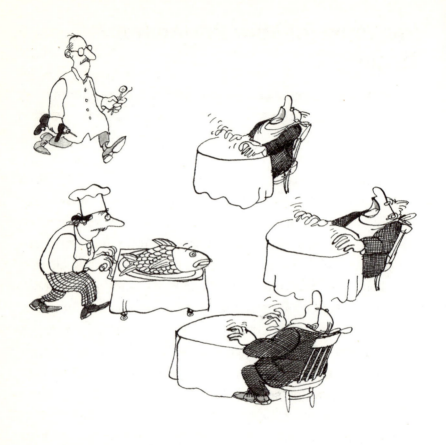

tooth. After the cleaning, avoid consuming things that are too cold or too hot, and stay away from sweet, sour, salty, and spicy foods. Rinsing with mildly warm saltwater will help to soothe the sensitive areas and help heal any small injuries sustained during the cleaning. Brushing and flossing may be a little painful for the first few days after the cleaning. Nevertheless, you should not stray from your oral hygiene routine. Another change you may notice is that the inside surfaces of the lower front teeth may feel different. This feeling is also temporary.

As you approach the date of the first stage of treatment, try not to imagine all of the detailed procedures. Instead imagine how you will be able to savor food after the restoration of your chewing apparatus. Look forward to enjoying pleasurable food and drink when you get home rather than feeling anxious about the treatments.

A major reconstruction can include a variety of stages. Sometimes crowns and fillings have to be repaired because they are fractured or have decayed around their margins, possibly as a result of insufficient oral hygiene. Because the margins of old crowns are often rough or overcontoured, plaque that cannot be removed by brushing or flossing builds up.

If the severity of your tooth and gum disease has advanced to the point that you have pockets around your teeth, the treatment will be more complex and take more time. The extent and duration of the restorative treatment depends on whether teeth have to be extracted before being replaced or whether gaps of missing teeth already exist at the onset of treatment. Even the kind of tooth replacement determines the extent of the treatment plan. If your teeth will be replaced by a simple prosthesis or denture, it will take less time than a fixed replacement, implant placement, or a combination thereof.

It can be time consuming to replace missing teeth with dental implants. Implants have to be placed in a healthy jaw, and two-stage protocols can entail a long healing period during which you will have to wear provisional teeth. After the healing process, the implants can be loaded with a crown or bridge. During the period of treatment your ability to chew, and therefore your ability to fully taste, depends on the type and composition of your provisional replacement. It will make a big difference whether the provisional restorations are cemented in place or whether they are removable. Always ask questions if you are unsure about what each treatment session will involve—such as what type of precautions you need to be aware of and how it will affect your chewing ability! The following chapters will explain different treatment steps in more detail. But first—a few suggestions to help make your eating limitations more enjoyable.

Astice Armoricaine con Riso Pilaf
Lobster Armoricaine with Rice Pilaf

Serves 6 as a main course
3 2-pound lobsters
2 cups Armoricaine sauce (see below)
2 tablespoons unsalted butter
2 tablespoons brandy
1 recipe rice pilaf (see below), mixed with ½ teaspoon curry powder
chopped flat-leaf parsley for garnish

Put the lobsters into a large pot of boiling water. When the water has returned to the boil, turn the heat to medium and boil the lobsters, covered, for 25 minutes. Remove the lobsters from the pot, drain, and let them cool.

Bend the lobsters backward until the shells crack; separate the tails from the bodies. Slit the shells on the underside of the tails with a knife or kitchen scissors. Remove the meat from the tails, in one piece if possible. Crack the claws and carefully remove the meat, preserving the shape of the claws if possible. Holding the knife at a 45-degree angle, slice the lobster tails into medallions. Refrigerate the lobster meat in a covered container.

Separate the lobster bodies from their shells. Remove and discard the stomach sac, which is right behind the eyes. Break up the lobster shells and bodies and use them to make the sauce.

To serve the lobster, heat 2 cups Armoricaine sauce in a small saucepan. Melt the butter in a skillet and gently heat the lobster meat just until it is warm. Pour on the brandy, warm it, and carefully ignite it. When the flames die out, add the hot sauce to the pan and combine well. Put a mound of rice pilaf in the center of a warmed platter and arrange the medallions of lobster and the claw meat decoratively around it. Spoon the sauce over all and sprinkle with chopped parsley.

For the Armoricaine sauce:

Makes about 1 quart
6 tablespoons olive oil
2 medium onions, chopped
1 carrot, chopped
2 celery ribs, chopped
1 garlic clove, chopped
Shells of at least 2 lobsters, broken up, and/or 6 cups shrimp shells, coarsely chopped
½ cup brandy
2 cups canned crushed tomatoes or 2 cups chopped canned peeled tomatoes with juice
2 quarts fish stock
2 large fresh thyme sprigs
salt
freshly ground pepper
⅛ teaspoon cayenne pepper
¼ cup flour

Heat the oil in a large soup pot over medium heat. Add the onion, carrot, celery, and garlic and cook for 20 minutes, stirring frequently. Add the lobster or shrimp shells and cook, stirring, for another 10 minutes. Pour on the brandy, heat it well, and carefully ignite it. Cook, tilting and rotating the pot, until the flames die out. Add the tomatoes, stir well, and simmer for 5 minutes. Add the stock, thyme, salt, pepper, and cayenne pepper and stir well. Bring to a boil, then reduce the heat and simmer, uncovered, for 15 minutes, stirring thoroughly every few minutes.

Skim ¼ cup of oil from the surface of the sauce and put it in a small saucepan. Heat it over medium heat. When it is bubbling, stir in the flour to form a roux and cook, stirring, for 3 or 4 minutes. Add a ladleful of hot sauce to the roux, whisk it until smooth, and then whisk in another ladleful of the hot liquid. Whisk the mixture until it is thick and smooth, then add it to the sauce in the pot. Stir in thoroughly and continue to simmer the sauce, uncovered, stirring frequently, for another 45 minutes.

Strain the sauce through a sieve over a large saucepan, shaking the sieve and pressing down on the solids to extract as much liquid as possible. The sauce will probably be too thin; boil it gently over medium heat until it has reduced and thickened. The sauce should be thick enough to coat the back of a spoon. Taste and adjust the seasoning.

For the rice pilaf:

Serves 6 as a first course or side dish
3½ cups chicken stock
¼ cup unsalted butter
1 small onion, cut in half
2 cups short-grain rice, preferably Italian, such as Carnaroli, Vialone, or Arborio
salt

Preheat oven to 350°F. Bring the chicken stock to a boil in a saucepan. Heat the butter in a Dutch oven over medium heat. Add the onion and cook until slightly softened but not browned, about 4 minutes. Add the rice, stir for a minute or 2 to coat with the butter, and add the boiling stock and some salt. Keep it boiling. Cover the Dutch oven with aluminum foil first, then the lid. Bake for 11 minutes without stirring. Remove the rice and spread it over a marble surface, a large tray, or a platter. It should cool off as quickly as possible. The rice pilaf is now ready. It will keep well in the refrigerator for up to 2 days. Before serving it, melt a little butter in a medium saucepan, add the rice, and stir gently with a fork. You can add ingredients as you please, for example, a teaspoon of curry powder, a little saffron, cooked mushrooms, or 3 cups of vegetables primavera. Add a little water if the rice is dry and/or sticking to the pan.

Wine notes

Italian: Terre di Tufo—Teruzzi & Puthod
American: Chardonnay—Callaway

Panini dell Harry's Bar

Harry's Bar Rolls
Makes 24

For the dough:
1¼-ounce package active dry yeast or 1 tablespoon brewer's yeast
1 cup lukewarm water or a little more if needed
3⅓ cups flour
2 tablespoons unsalted butter at room temperature
2 teaspoons salt
2 teaspoons sugar
¾ cup unsalted butter, cut into bits and kept chilled (for kneading)

The easiest way to make the dough for these rolls is in the food processor. Sprinkle the yeast over a cup of lukewarm water. Let it sit for 5 minutes, then stir to blend. Put the flour, butter, salt, and sugar in the bowl of a processor fitted with a steel blade. Turn on the motor and, after 30 seconds, pour the yeast mixture through the feeding tube and process it for a minute or so. If the dough does not form a ball, add lukewarm water a tablespoon at a time just until the dough forms a ball.

Turn the dough out of the processor, knead it for a minute, and put it in a bowl. Let it rest for 30 minutes, covered with a damp kitchen towel. Spread the bits of butter for kneading on a piece of wax paper and leave them at room temperature.

If you want to mix the dough by hand, rinse a large mixing bowl with hot water and dry it. Sprinkle the yeast over the luke-

warm water in the warmed bowl and let it sit for 5 minutes. Stir to blend, then add the flour, butter, salt, and sugar. Mix everything together, at first with a fork and then with your hands, to form a soft dough. Knead for a minute or 2 to blend thoroughly. Shape the dough into a ball and leave it in the bowl, covered with a damp kitchen towel, for 30 minutes. Spread the bits of butter for kneading on a piece of wax paper and leave them at room temperature.

Put a cup of flour on the work surface near you and dust the surface and your rolling pin lightly but frequently to keep the dough from sticking when you knead or roll it.

Knead the dough for a minute or 2. Using a well-floured rolling pin, roll the dough into a rectangle, approximately 10 by 15 inches, with the short side toward you. Sprinkle the bits of butter over the top two-thirds of the dough, leaving a good 1-inch margin of dough. Fold the dough in thirds like a business letter, starting from the bottom. Press on the edges of the dough to seal the butter in. Be sure the butter is enclosed in the folded dough.

Turn the dough so the narrow edge is toward you, roll it out into a rectangle again, and fold it again in thirds. Wrap the dough in the damp kitchen towel and refrigerate it for 30 minutes.

Remove the dough from the refrigerator and roll, fold, and turn it 2 more times. Cover it with the damp towel and refrigerate it for another 30 minutes.

Remove the dough from the refrigerator and roll, fold, and turn it 2 more times. Cover it with the damp towel and refrigerate it for another 30 minutes.

Roll the dough into a 12-by-14-inch rectangle. Cut the rectangle in half lengthwise. Working with half the dough at a time, brush the surface with a little water and, using your fingers, form a long cylinder of dough by rolling the strip of dough over itself lengthwise. Repeat with the other half of the dough. Cut each cylinder into 12 pieces and put them, cut side up, on buttered baking sheets. Do not crowd the rolls; leave 1½ inches around each one. Cover the baking sheets with damp kitchen towels and put the rolls in a warm place to rise for 2 hours.

Preheat the oven to 400°F.

Bake the rolls in the upper third of the oven until they are golden, about 25 minutes. Let them cool briefly. Serve warm, at room temperature, or briefly reheated in a 400°F oven. These rolls can be frozen. To reheat, place the frozen rolls in a 400°F oven for 5 minutes.

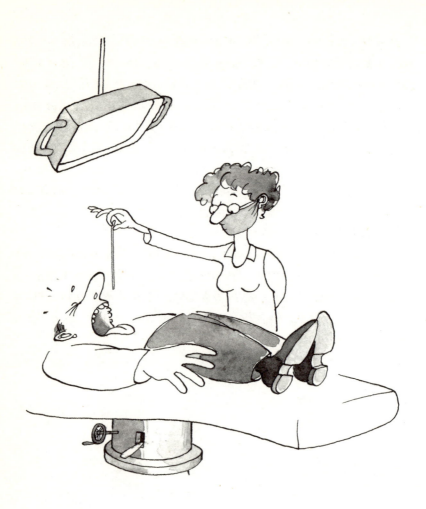

Simple Tooth Extraction

If your dentist's prognosis for your teeth is hopeless, your first stage of treatment will involve extracting the hopeless teeth. As you give yourself over to this plan, you may feel nervous and ambiguous even though you know it is for the best. As you sit there, a prisoner of the dental chair, you brace yourself for the most painful part: the shot. OUCHHHH—there it is. The comforting hand of the dental assistant on one shoulder does not lessen the pain, although it does reassure you that everything will be okay in the hands of these professionals.

Soon you feel like the left half of your face has grown to monstrous proportions and is being controlled by an entity outside your body. It does not even seem to be part of your body. A cottony feeling of numbness crawls behind your left ear and eye. Again, the supporting hands are there. They wrap around your head, preventing both sides of your face from drifting apart.

With forceps the dentist separates the broken remnants of the tooth from the jawbone without breaking it. The operation has been successful! After placement of the gauze, the assistant instructs you on your aftercare and follow-up and answers any questions you might have. You are advised to wait until the numbness wears off before eating. How long it will be will depend on the rate of metabolism. One more thing: The soothing voice warns, DO NOT SMOKE. You better not protest—instead, sit there and do as you're told!

Initial postoperative meals, you are told, cannot include any foods containing crust or small seeds. During the new growth of blood vessels, cells, and oral mucosa, special eating guidelines have to be followed. This process takes a few days. After a few months the cavity left by the wound will be filled with growing bone.

Milk products of any kind should not be consumed for 3 days because they degrade, or rot, in the oral environment and produce compounds that can destroy the blood clot.

Smoking should definitely be avoided because it is the worst enemy of the healing process. Nicotine causes capillaries to constrict, which prevents the critical passage of fluid with all of its nourishing and immunologic properties. Dangerous complications could result.

Recurring pain and a bad odor are signs that the healing process has been disrupted, and these signs prompt an urgent visit to the dentist.

You have been listening attentively to all of this advice, and you bravely vow to obey all instructions. It is for your own good!

Spezzatino con Carciofi
Veal Stew with Artichokes

The name of this stew is derived from the word spezzare—to break—and the stew is traditionally made from "broken veal," the trimmings from veal shanks or chops. Spezzatini are made with very few ingredients, very lightly seasoned, and they are surprisingly delicious. After making this one with artichokes, try some variations of your own, using, for example, mushrooms, asparagus, or potatoes—but don't be tempted to add a lot of extra seasoning. Simplicity is the secret to this dish.

Serves 6 as a main course
2 pounds boneless veal shoulder, cut into 1-inch cubes
salt
freshly ground pepper
flour for dredging
2 tablespoons unsalted butter
2 tablespoons olive oil
1 medium onion, chopped
2 celery ribs, chopped
1 garlic clove, minced
1 cup dry white wine
warm stock or water if needed

For the artichokes:
6 large artichokes
2 tablespoons olive oil
1 garlic clove, crushed

Season the veal pieces with salt and pepper, dredge them in flour, and shake off any excess. Heat the butter and oil in a large skillet over medium heat, and brown the meat on all sides, in batches if necessary. Add the onion, celery, and garlic to the pan, stir them in, and sauté for just a minute or 2. Turn up the heat to high, add the wine to the skillet, and boil it briskly for a minute or 2, scraping up the brown bits from the bottom of the pan. Turn the heat down to medium-low and season with salt and pepper. Cover the pan and cook the mixture gently for about 45 minutes, adding a little warm stock or water from time to time if needed.

Meanwhile, prepare the artichokes as directed on page 32. Heat the oil and garlic in a skillet over medium heat, add the sliced artichokes, and cook, stirring frequently, until they are tender—about 8 to 10 minutes. Remove the garlic and stir the artichokes into the veal. Continue to simmer the stew until the meat is very tender—about 45 minutes. Serve with rice pilaf (page 52).

Wine notes
Italian: Chianti—Saccardi
American: Merlot—Matanzas Creek

Surgical Tooth Extraction

Teeth cannot always be easily extracted with forceps. Sometimes the gum around the tooth has to be cut into in order to remove the tooth or its remnants from the bone. Then of course the wound has to be sutured. For the first few days after such a procedure, abstinence from solid foods or minimal food intake may be the most soothing. If wisdom teeth were removed, soup or other liquid foods may be recommended for a few days. Use of a straw may be necessary at first. As with the simple pulling of teeth with forceps, milk products of any kind should be avoided, as should anything containing hard elements such as crust or seeds. Alcohol may be consumed in small amounts—after all, a suffering person should not be deprived of this comforter. Again, nicotine must be avoided, especially during the first 36 hours after the procedure. Even coffee should be avoided, especially espresso.

Remember: Even with a closed wound, a successful healing process needs at least 3 days! Furthermore, sutured wounds may not be fully closed or they may not be closed tightly because of inflammation. Sutures can loosen or break because of the pressure caused by swelling. In such a case, the reopened wound is especially prone to inflammation. Interferences in the healing process will not only extend the healing time, but may worsen the end result because the healing tissue is not able to rebuild properly. In esthetic areas of the oral cavity, unsightly scars from improper healing can lead to extensive reconstruction procedures to restore the natural char-

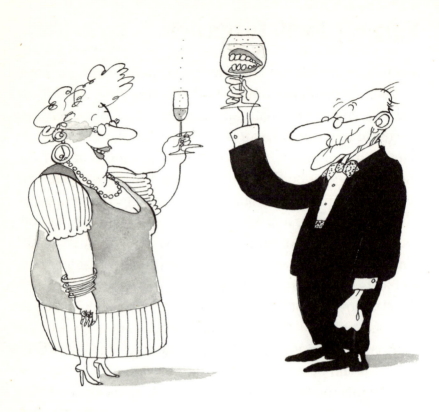

acteristics. Defective healing can also cause critical complications, especially after removal of the lower wisdom teeth. Behind the wisdom teeth in the lower jaw are blood vessels and nerves. In addition, inflammation of the lower jaw is hard to treat.

Let us backtrack to the subject of alcohol. One glass of the preferred alcoholic beverage should have a sufficiently positive effect. If you prefer wine it is best to stay away from those that are acidic. Wines with high acidic contents—such as the Rheingau Riesling wines—will badly damage the teeth.

We sought the advice of one of the most prestigious sommeliers in Europe—Mr Bernd Kreis from Stuttgart, Germany:

Every wine has several acids. There are 10 different acids in wine, each of them with different levels of sourness, as well as different tastes. Malic acid is one of the most acidic acids and can be mainly found in unripe grapes and in grapes from vineyards with an overly high production rate per grapevine. In general, wines harvested with riper grapes and distinguished as high quality are less acidic; the acids of a high-quality wine are milder than those of wine made from poor-quality grapes. Besides the quality of the grapes, there are two other factors of importance. When reviewing white wines, the geographic origin of the wine is important. Wines from warm areas are less acidic than those from cooler areas. Even though wines from cooler climates are more elegant and distinct, they stimulate the sensitive cervical areas of the teeth as much as they do the taste buds, but in an opposing manner. The type of wine is another determinant of the level of acidity. For example, with Chardonnay, a technique called malolactic fermentation is used to reduce the

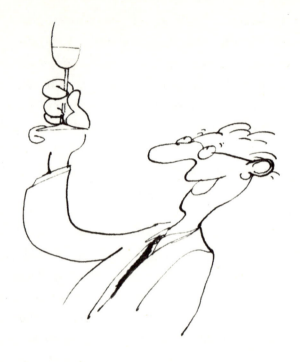

acidity. After the alcoholic fermentation process is finished, lactic acid bacteria convert the aggressive malic acid into carbonic acid and mild lactic acid. In general, all oak-aged Chardonnays undergo malolactic fermentation and can therefore be recommended for people with tooth problems. The most famous wines of this kind come from California, Oregon, and Washington State. Chardonnay is a real cosmopolitan; it has similar characteristics from vineyards all over the world. Therefore, one can choose a Chardonnay from this broad spectrum without worry. Those who like fruity fresh white wines may also choose a

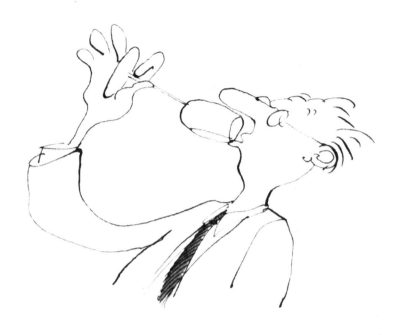

Sauvignon blanc, but please choose one that originates from a warm region, such as California or Chile. The more acidic ones from France or New Zealand should remain on the shelf. Viognier is a great alternative. It is as fruity as Sauvignon blanc and it is less acidic. Chenin blanc is always worth a try. With this wine you should select from warmer regions, such as California, Mexico, and South Africa. The Chenins from the French Loire Valley should be reserved for the period after recovery. Rieslings are becoming more and more popular, especially those from Germany and Austria. However, Rieslings from these areas are

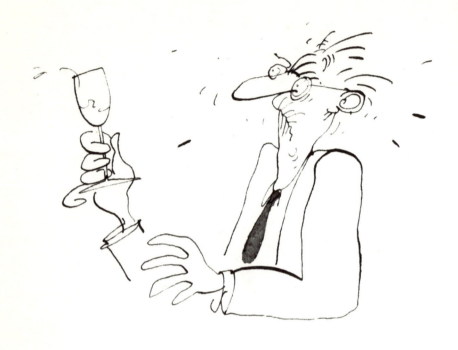

very acidic despite their fruity, sweet taste. Patients would be safer with a Riesling from Oregon or Australia, since those wines have a lower level of acidity. Sweet wines such as noble late-harvest wines, Sauternes, and Vin Santo should also remain in the dental patient's wine cellar. These delicious drops are pressed with overly ripe and dried grapes, which not only have concentrated sweetness but also high levels of acid. Sparkling wines such as Champagne should be avoided as well. Patients may look forward to a glass or two after the healing process. These wines generally contain a high level of acid, which is intensified by the carbonation.

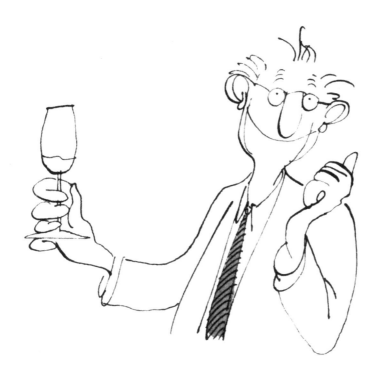

Red wines are problematic, not because of the acidity but rather because of the pigment and tannins. The level of pigment and tannins depends on several factors, the largest of which is the origin. In warm and sunny regions the grapes protect themselves through intensified color, tannins, and a thick layer of skin. We can therefore conclude that grapes grown with a lot of sun contribute a higher level of tannins and more intense color. The dye discolors the teeth and the tannins attack the enamel. Real killers are Cabernets and blends of Syrah, Grenache, and Mourvedre. Even though they guarantee a wonderful flavor, they

can be torturous to the teeth. Cooler climates, such as Washington State and Oregon, produce wines containing a lower degree of pigment and tannins. Wines made from Pinot Noir grapes are ideal. Wonderful Pinot Noirs come from France (Burgundy region), South Africa, and New Zealand. The German and Italian Pinot Noirs from Alto Adige and Trentino deserve credit as well. By the way, tannins and pigments weaken through the ripening process; therefore it is always better to choose a ripe wine.

Salmone Agli Zucchini

Poached Salmon with Zucchini Sauce

Serves 6 as a main course

For the sauce:

2 cups water
4 medium zucchini (about 1½ pounds) cut into eighths
1 medium onion, sliced
5 tablespoons red wine vinegar
freshly ground white pepper
⅛ teaspoon cayenne pepper
2 tablespoons olive oil
1 celery rib, chopped
1 medium onion, chopped
2 tablespoons unsalted butter
2 tablespoons flour
1 teaspoon curry powder
1 cup milk
salt

For the salmon:

1 cup dry white wine
2 cups water plus extra as needed
1 tablespoon fresh lemon juice
1 celery rib, coarsely chopped
1 onion, coarsely chopped
1 carrot, coarsely chopped

1 bay leaf
salt
freshly ground pepper
6 center-cut salmon fillets or 2 pounds salmon fillet cut into 6 serving pieces

Prepare the sauce: *Bring the water, zucchini, sliced onion, 2 tablespoons of the vinegar, white pepper, and cayenne pepper to a boil in a large saucepan. Cover the pot, reduce the heat slightly, and boil until the zucchini and onion are soft—15 to 20 minutes.*

Meanwhile, heat the olive oil in a small skillet over medium-low heat. Add the chopped celery and onion and cook until the vegetables are soft and golden—about 10 minutes. Add the remaining vinegar and boil for another 2 minutes. Add this mixture to the zucchini. Using a food processor fitted with a steel blade, or a blender, puree the vegetables and liquid until smooth.

Melt the butter in a large saucepan over medium heat. Add the flour and curry powder and whisk for 2 or 3 minutes. Gradually whisk in the milk, then add the zucchini mixture and whisk until completely blended. Boil over medium-high heat, stirring frequently, until slightly thickened—about 10 minutes. Season to taste and strain through a fine sieve into a saucepan. Keep warm over low heat.

Prepare the salmon: *Bring the wine, water, lemon juice, celery, onion, carrot, bay leaf, salt, and pepper to a boil in a deep skillet and boil for 5 minutes. Strain the mixture and return the liquid to the skillet. Bring this poaching liquid to a boil and add the salmon. Turn down the heat and maintain a steady simmer. If the* *fish is not covered by the poaching liquid, carefully turn it over after about 4 minutes. Poach the salmon just until it flakes—5 to 7 minutes. Using a slotted spatula, put the salmon on a heated platter and spoon the zucchini sauce on top. Serve with fried zucchini.*

For the fried zucchini:
Serves 6 as a side dish
olive oil or sunflower oil for frying
1 cup flour
1 teaspoon salt
freshly ground pepper
8 small zucchini (about 2 pounds), sliced crosswise ⅛-inch thick

Heat an inch of oil in a large skillet until it is very hot.
While the oil is heating, put the flour, salt, and some pepper in a paper bag. Add the zucchini slices and shake the bag. Pour the contents of the bag into a sieve, and shake to remove excess flour. Drop a handful of zucchini slices into the oil, being careful not to overcrowd them in the pan, and fry, turning them until they are golden. Transfer to paper towels to drain. Repeat with the remaining zucchini. Season with salt and serve immediately.

Wine notes
Italian: Gavi—La Scolca
American: Chardonnay Reserve—Mondavi

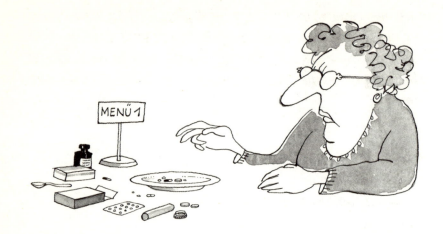

Antibiotics

The removal of the molar on the upper right may have necessitated a more complex procedure than expected. Cutting, drilling, and suturing put more stress on your already compromised tissues; therefore, your dentist will probably prescribe an antibiotic as a preventive measure or, in the case of secondary sinus inflammation, as treatment for an infection.

Your dentist will emphasize that the antibiotic treatment should not be curtailed before the complete course is finished! An antibiotic kills bacteria within the body and prevents their growth and multiplication. If the antibiotic treatment is stopped too early, resistant bacteria will survive that cannot be killed as effectively with the same antibiotic the next time an illness is present. Therefore, following the prescription protocol is very important.

A variety of antibiotics exist, some of which may cause digestive problems. Besides killing the bacteria causing the inflammation in your oral cavity, the antibiotic also kills some of the natural bacteria in the intestine. Because these bacteria contribute to a healthy digestive system, their destruction may result in some digestive disturbance. To avoid any complications, such as an intestinal infection, you need to adjust your eating habits as soon as you start taking the first dose. You will have to eat small portions of food at each meal, washed down with lots of fluid. This is not to say that you have to reduce the amount of food you usually consume in a day, just that each meal has to be small—therefore, you may end up eating several small meals instead of three larger meals. Some patients have reported that an additional intake of fillers, such as a mixture of linseeds, oat bran, and wheat bran can be helpful.

I often see patients who are in a weakened physical and mental state because their constant dental pain has prevented them from taking in adequate nutrients and has necessitated the continuous use of pain medication. You cannot withstand a dental procedure and antibiotic treatment in such a state. Special diet measures can help prevent such conditions beforehand. The intake of sufficient fluids and nutrients is critical before and after a dental procedure.

Many dentists suggest staying away from alcohol while taking antibiotics. With very few exceptions, however, the antibiotics on the market today are not affected by alcohol consumption. In other words: Nothing speaks against one glass of red wine to comfort the injured soul. We are talking about alcohol in moderation, of course. The rule "more is better" does not apply in this case. One glass of wine with dinner might be considered a medically supported dose.

Pollo con Verdure

Chicken with Vegetables

Serves 6 as a main course
¾ pound carrots
1 medium zucchini
2 celery ribs
1 red bell pepper
1 green bell pepper
2 large artichokes, trimmed and sliced (see page 32)
6 chicken breasts and/or thighs and drumsticks
salt
freshly ground pepper
flour for dredging
¼ cup olive oil
¾ cup dry white wine

Cut the carrots, zucchini, celery, and bell peppers into 1-by-½-inch strips. Set a large bowl of ice water on a surface next to the stove.

Blanch the vegetables: Bring a large pot of water to a boil over high heat. Add the carrot pieces and boil them for about 30 seconds after the water returns to a full boil. Remove the carrots with a slotted spoon or strainer and submerge them in the bowl of ice water. Repeat with the zucchini pieces and then with the celery pieces, cooking each until they are bright green—about 30 seconds. Blanch the red and green peppers for about 30 seconds. Repeat with the artichoke slices, cooking them for

1 minute. Drain the vegetables, pat them dry, and set them aside. Preheat the oven to 375°F.

Pat the chicken pieces dry, season them with salt and pepper and dredge them in flour, shaking off any excess. Heat the oil in a heavy skillet over medium-high heat. Add the chicken pieces and cook them, in batches if necessary, turning them once, until they are golden brown and crisp on both sides—about 15 minutes. Remove the chicken from the pan and put it in a 14-inch oval or round dish.

Pour off all but 1 tablespoon of fat from the pan, add the wine, and bring it to a boil over high heat, scraping up the brown bits from the bottom of the pan. Add the vegetables and simmer the mixture, stirring constantly, for 2 to 3 minutes. Pour the vegetables and juices over the chicken, cover the dish (with foil if it has no lid), and put it in the oven. Bake for about 30 minutes, until the chicken is tender and the juices run clear, with no tinge of pink, when it is pierced with a sharp knife. Taste and adjust the seasoning.

Serve the chicken with one spoonful of vegetables and one of pan juices.

Wine notes
Italian: Merlot—Livio Felluga
American: Merlot—Matanzas Creek

Provisional Teeth

When your natural teeth have to be filed down to prepare for a crown or to serve as an anchor for a bridge, they lose their protective enamel layer. The dentin underneath is then exposed. You may have experienced how an exposed and filed tooth peg can hurt when stimulated by triggers such as temperature and pressure stimuli. The exposed dentin is an open wound, with thousands of freshly cut nerve canals that must be protected. To prevent bacteria from finding their way into the nerve canals and the inner part of the tooth where they could cause severe pain, nerve death, and suppurative inflammation around the tooth, the prepared tooth is fitted with a protective provisional tooth until the final tooth is ready. A provisional restoration can be fabricated best on a plaster cast of the prepared tooth. You may still experience sensitivity with the provisional tooth in place because sensitive areas near the root that are normally covered by gum may be exposed.

Especially with extensive bridgework, tension and pain can occur because of the strong forces used when eating. Therefore your dentist should use a metal framework for the provisional restoration rather than a temporary resin composite. A stronger frame will allow you to eat hard and tough foods without danger. The provisional restoration is only a temporary solution, but in many cases, it will be the pattern for the final restoration. With good patient feedback, the dentist can address any patient complaints before the dental technician fabricates the final restoration. If you have difficulty eating with your provisional restoration, tell

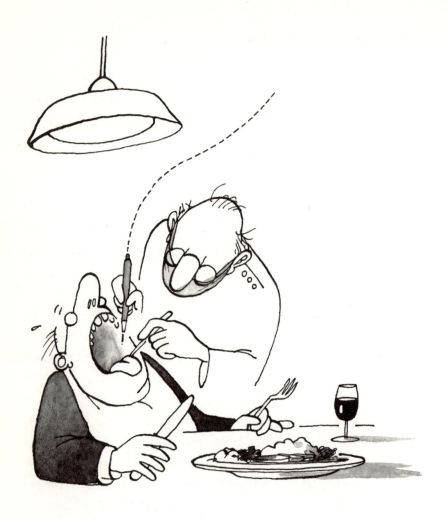

your dentist right away. Don't suffer needlessly. The following story will convince you of that.

Almost 20 years ago I had a patient who was in need of extensive dental restoration. This patient, a very kind man, spoke again and again about the beauty of his homeland, Sardinia. After many appointments at my practice, he succeeded in persuading me to spend my vacation in Sardinia. I placed his provisional restorations just before I left, so that his gums would be healed by the time I returned.

It happened that my patient was going to be in Sardinia visiting his family at around the same time as my vacation. He found a place for me to stay, with an older couple who grew wine grapes on their farm.

The evening before my departure, the farmer invited all of us to a big dinner of roasted baby goat. The meat tasted fabulous, although it did require a powerful biting armamentarium. As I chewed with all of my might, I glanced at each member of the dinner party. I was astonished at what I saw. The farmer appeared to be toothless and yet did not show any signs of discomfort while trying to chew the meat. Even his wife, who wore dentures made by the local dental technician, savored the meal without any sign of difficulty. Furthermore, my patient's mother, a butcher's wife, joyfully ate the meal with her four or five remaining teeth. The only one who ate quietly and slowly at this happy dinner table was my patient—with the provisional restorations made by me! It was obvious how hard and painful it was for this man to bite and chew the food. I started to feel doubt, which could be described as a professional identity crisis.

What a sight! There were people eating joyfully with at most a few teeth left in their mouths, while my patient, who had the "benefits" of modern dentistry, suffered through the meal trying to eat with difficulty. If I had not known that he would be getting permanent crowns and bridges within a few weeks, with which he would be able to bite through any tough meat, I would have had to have answered the question of the deeper purpose of our profession with a larger amount of Sardinian wine. That evening we laughed at numerous jokes, primarily at my expense. I could only think to the next year, when my patient's dental treatment would be completed and any culinary challenge could be mastered with ease.

My patient, who still uses our services regularly—almost 20 years later—is still laughing about that story. If I may add: He is laughing with the same crowns.

Piccata di Vitello al Limone

Veal Scallops with Lemon

About veal piccata (scaloppini) in general: Be careful not to overcook the veal. Never dredge the scaloppini in flour until you are just ready to cook them; if you do it ahead of time, the flour becomes damp, and the meat won't brown properly. Make sure that the oil is very hot when you put the scaloppini in the pan. Cook them very rapidly, just until the edges are lightly browned, which should take 2 minutes or less on each side.

Serves 6 as a main course
flour for dredging
1½ pounds boneless veal round or leg, sliced ¼-inch thick and pounded thin for scaloppini
salt
freshly ground pepper
3 to 6 tablespoons olive oil
½ cup chicken stock
¼ cup fresh lemon juice
3 tablespoons unsalted butter
2 tablespoons finely chopped flat-leaf parsley

Preheat the oven to 200°F and put a platter in to warm. Put a small pile of flour on a work surface next to the stove.

Trim the veal scallops so they are all approximately the same size, and season them with salt and pepper. Heat 2 to 3 table-

spoons of the oil to sizzling in your largest skillet. Dip 6 to 8 veal pieces in the flour, shake off the excess, and add the meat to the pan. Cook as rapidly as possible—not more than 2 minutes on each side. Transfer the meat to the warmed serving dish in the oven. Repeat until all the meat is done, adding more oil to the pan as needed. Pour off the oil from the pan, raise the heat, and add the chicken stock. Boil, scraping up all the brown bits from the bottom of the pan. Add the lemon juice, season with salt and pepper, and boil for another minute or so. Remove the pan from the heat, add the butter, and whisk until blended. Stir in the parsley and pour the sauce over the veal. Serve immediately.

Gum Surgery

The treatments for gum disease in the past would be considered barbaric by today's standards. Not too long ago, diseased gums were cut or even burned off, probably not too different from medieval dentistry! Today the treatment of severe gum disease may result in partial loss of the gum, but the loss is not permanent. The regeneration of gum tissue is part of the overall treatment plan, especially in the esthetic zone that shows when you talk, smile, and laugh. And laugh again you will, confidently, when it is all over. More good news: this treatment does not interfere with your ability to taste.

As we have already mentioned, gum disease due to plaque buildup and the resulting inflammation of the gums, or even the destruction of the supporting tissue and fibers that connect the tooth to the bone, occurs mainly in adults after the age of 30. In younger patients, gum disease is usually due to a compromised immune system or a genetic disease.

Proper treatment always begins with a thorough analysis of the contributing factors. When patients are aware of these factors, they are motivated to take steps to fight the disease and maintain their health through hygienic interventions as instructed by the dental hygienist. The hygienist will begin the treatment by removing the plaque above and under the gum line. After the cleaning, the inflamed gum will shrink, exposing the sensitive cervical areas of the teeth. These areas may continue to be sensitive throughout the healing process. As described earlier, rinse with lightly salted warm water. The

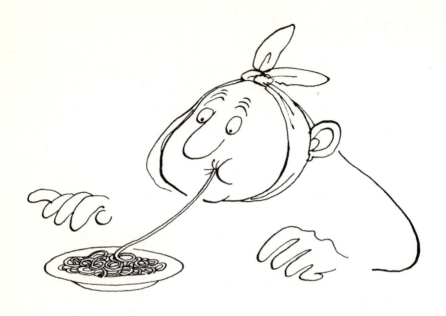

rinse will support the healing process more than those chemical rinses that can be found in advertisements.

After the gum has healed, the lost tissue and existing pockets will have to be reconstructed. In most cases, the treatment can be done in stages, so that only part of your mouth is treated at each appointment. Nevertheless, you have to adjust your eating habits to this situation.

The following aftercare guidelines, some of which have been mentioned throughout this book as friendly reminders, apply to any dental treatment: Do not eat before the numbness wears off! Do not consume any milk products for 3 days! Do not eat any foods with small seeds or with a sharp crust! Stay away from hot and cold, sweet and sour, and heavily seasoned foods! Nicotine is absolutely forbidden! As explained in a previous chapter, nicotine reduces the capillary blood flow and thus compromises healing. In addition, it inhibits the development of specific defense cells, so that the risk for re-infection is increased 20 times, according to scientific research. It is best to use this opportunity to quit smoking altogether.

Last, after eating anything, rinse your mouth to flush away loose food particles. And, at least once within a 24-hour period, you must thoroughly brush and floss your teeth. Consult your dental hygienist regarding the proper way to brush and floss after gum surgery.

In general, the healing process after gum treatment takes longer than generally expected. While you may not remember exactly how many weeks ago the sutures were removed, your body is busy regenerating destroyed tissue in deep areas and reshaping the surface. Your body can accomplish this amazing feat only if you provide the necessary nutrition and oral hygiene. Aside from the limitations listed above, do not deprive your taste buds of delicious food and drink—instead, nurture your mental and physical well-being with healthy and pleasurable foods.

Risotto alla Milanese

Saffron Risotto

This risotto is the classic accompaniment to ossobuco. Some add a little marrow to this recipe for its unique flavor and richness. If you add marrow, use only 1 tablespoon of butter.

Serves 6 as a first course
½ teaspoon saffron threads or ⅛ teaspoon powdered saffron, dissolved in ½ cup hot stock
2 tablespoons veal marrow (optional)
1 recipe risotto parmigiano (see page 29)

Prepare the risotto as directed. If you are using marrow, add it to the sautéed onions before you add the rice. Add the saffron stock after 15 minutes and finish the risotto as directed.

For the marrow:
2 to 3 pounds veal marrow bones
1 onion, cut into squares
1 bay leaf
1 teaspoon salt

Put all of the ingredients into a 3-quart pot. Add 7 to 8 cups of cold water or enough to barely cover the bones. Bring the water to a boil, partially cover the pot, reduce the heat to medium-low, and cook the bones for 2½ to 3 hours. Pour off the stock through a strainer and use it to make the risotto.

Remember: Push or scoop the marrow from the center of the bones and add it to the onion mixture before you add the rice.

Wine notes

Italian: Nebbiolo d'Alba—Giacosa
 Chianti—Vigorello, San Felice
American: Zinfandel—Lytton Springs

The Joy of Dental Implants

The ability to replace lost teeth with permanent, fixed replications of the natural teeth has been a dream come true for dentists and patients. To regain the pleasure of eating, tasting, talking, doing everything your healthy mouth could once do—enhances life in general.

If you have or have had dentures, you know what it feels like to look in the bathroom mirror with your dentures in place and what it feels like to look at your reflection after you have removed the dentures for cleaning. Daily you have to face the gaps, the golden tooth stumps, the unsupported facial contours that no one but you ever sees. For many people, part of growing old is getting this third set of—removable—teeth. The TV commercials that show smiling denture wearers selling adhesive fail to mention all of the disadvantages of removable prostheses, including the difficulty in cleaning them or the limitations in tasting food, and some people get the wrong idea.

A patient recently told me about his 11-year-old son who had lost both central incisors in a bicycle fall and had thought that he would now grow his third set of teeth! The misconception probably came from TV commercials. Fortunately, artificial teeth are not what they used to be. Now the manufactured teeth are implanted in the jawbone, whereby these realistic prosthetic teeth integrate into the bone and remain there permanently. Implant-supported crowns or bridges in any combination permanently replace all necessary teeth.

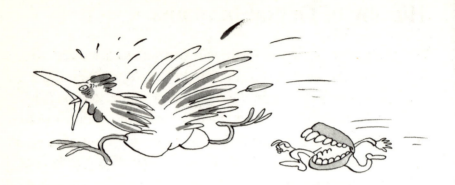

Three decades ago, implant dentistry had a bad reputation among dental researchers. Conscientious scientists did not support such treatment, because the longevity of implants was limited and the failure rate high. In case of failure, patients had to deal with drastic consequences involving the jawbone; furthermore, if the implant failed, their only option was to have a removable denture. A few years later the Swedish scientist Professor Per-Ingvar Brånemark revolutionized dentistry.

As a researcher in bone growth during the 1960s, Brånemark found, by accident, that titanium could integrate into bone and could only be separated by applying a strong force. He had been implanting microscopes with a steel casing into live bone and retrieving them once the project was over. One day, the microscopes had integrated into the bone so tightly that they could not be removed without removing the surrounding bone. He discovered that the English manufacturer of this particular microscope used titanium casings instead of steel. The result was an accidental fusion of the titanium casing with the bone tissue around it. This finding was the birth of the titanium implant.

The applications of this discovery spread throughout all of medicine. But it was not until the late 1980s that its use in dentistry achieved predictable, reliable results. Meanwhile, scientific research has shown that implants can last more than 30 years, with a low failure rate, between 3% and 5%.

Since the late 1980s, further developments in implant dentistry have made it possible for patients to laugh and smile without anyone noticing that the teeth are not real. Even professional experts have a hard time identifying implants apart from natural teeth. Besides the cosmetic benefits, patients can enjoy eating their favorite foods as much as they did when they had their own teeth.

As is usual in life, high quality comes with a high price and a high level of commitment—not only financial but temporal. It can be a hard journey from losing your teeth to having a final implant-supported prosthesis in place. After the implant placement, provisional teeth are worn while the bone heals around the implants. This process can be compared to a trip through a harsh desert to a green paradise full of forgotten treasures—what you thought you had lost along with your teeth greets you on the other side.

Patients who have not attained their full growth have to go through a longer journey, unfortunately. Let us go back to the 11-year-old boy who lost his two front teeth. If he does not want to sacrifice the neighboring teeth for a bridge, he will have to wear a temporary prosthesis until his jawbone is fully grown, at which time implants can be placed. The long wait is worth it, though. After 10 years, he will forget about the negative experiences associated with the treatment, and he will be relieved that his neighboring teeth were spared.

The loss of posterior teeth is not as bad, although your quality of life will be worse during the surgical phase of implant placement in this area, which entails suturing so the tissue can heal.

The period of healing is the most critical phase of treatment, especially when implants are placed in less-stable bone. The upper jawbone is less dense and softer than the lower jawbone, so it takes longer for the implants to fully integrate.

The duration of the healing period depends on many factors and must be determined for each patient. In some cases, it is possible to load the implants right away or after a short healing period. But if the bone has to be built up, or if the bone is unusually soft, the healing time may be longer. Just remember that your body took 8 years to develop your first set of teeth, so be patient and give your dentist, and your body, the necessary time to achieve success.

For patients who have lost all of their teeth, and for whom complete acrylic resin dentures dampen any pleasure of eating, the decision to have dental implants can mean a temporary worsening of the quality of life following implant placement. With a mouth full of sutures and swollen tissue, a period of rest is necessary; any stresses and interferences in the healing process need to be avoided. It is best to prepare for this event by having your kitchen stocked with ingredients for meals that will be kind to your healing wounds and delicious to your palate.

Another reminder: Even though milk products are soft, they are forbidden during the initial healing phase! Foods that are crusty or have hard, small particles that can loosen and migrate into the wound should be avoided. These rules apply throughout the entire healing period, even when you are using a provisional prosthesis (with a soft lining), and when you are able to eat more normal foods.

Also, and this is the last reminder: Stay away from nicotine as long as possible! Avoid hot and cold foods and beverages! Avoid strong coffee, which hinders the circulation and therefore wound healing! And avoid acidic or very spicy foods and beverages!

When your time of suffering is nearing the end, thanks to the right treatment, hygiene, and eating habits, the promised paradise is visible at the horizon, and a new life awaits you! You will once again have fixed teeth to bite and chew with. Think about all of those tantalizing foods that you can savor fully! One who has not lost an invaluable treasure cannot appreciate what it feels like to find it again, whole and unharmed. You will know this feeling, and you will rejoice!

Tagliolini con Funghi alla Cipriani
Egg Pasta with Wild Mushrooms

Serves 6 as a first course or 4 as a main course
2 tablespoons unsalted butter
2 cups thinly sliced shiitake or other wild mushrooms
1 small garlic clove, chopped
2 tablespoons finely chopped flat-leaf parsley
½ cup dry white wine
½ cup heavy cream
½ cup tomato sauce (see below)
salt
freshly ground pepper
¾ pound dried tagliolini
3 tablespoons freshly grated Parmesan cheese, plus extra to pass at the table
1 cup béchamel sauce (see below)

Bring a large pot of water to a boil.

Melt the butter in a large skillet over medium heat. Add the mushrooms and cook until they are tender and the mushroom liquid has evaporated—about 6 to 8 minutes. Add the garlic and parsley and cook for 30 seconds. Add the white wine and cook for 2 minutes. Add the heavy cream and bring it to a boil. Reduce the heat, add the tomato sauce, and simmer for 2 minutes more. Taste and season with salt and freshly ground pepper.

Preheat the broiler.

Add a tablespoon of salt to the boiling water, cook the pasta for 2 minutes or until al dente, and drain well in a colander.

Toss the pasta with the mushroom mixture, add 2 tablespoons of the Parmesan, and toss well. Spread the pasta evenly in a warmed shallow baking dish, spread on the béchamel, and top with the remaining Parmesan. Broil 3 inches from the heat source for 2 to 3 minutes, turning the pan as necessary to brown evenly. Serve immediately, passing around a small bowl of grated Parmesan cheese.

For the tomato sauce:

Makes about 2½ cups
¼ cup olive oil
¼ cup minced onion
1 28-ounce can crushed Italian plum tomatoes or whole tomatoes, chopped, with juices
salt
freshly ground pepper
1 bay leaf
1 tablespoon finely chopped fresh basil leaves

Heat the oil in a saucepan over medium heat. Add the onion and cook it, stirring frequently, until it is wilted—about 4 minutes. Add the tomatoes, salt, pepper, and bay leaf and heat to boiling.

Reduce the heat to low and simmer, uncovered, for about 30 minutes, stirring frequently. Stir in the chopped basil and simmer for 5 minutes longer. Strain the mixture through a colander set over a bowl.

For the béchamel sauce:

Makes 2 cups
¼ cup unsalted butter
¼ cup flour
2 cups milk
salt
freshly ground white pepper

Melt the butter in the top of a double boiler or in a heavy-bottomed saucepan over low heat. Whisk in the flour and cook gently without browning, stirring constantly, for 4 or 5 minutes. Take the pan off the heat and vigorously whisk in the milk. Cold milk will whisk in smoothly if you remove the pan from the heat. When the sauce is well blended, return it to the stove and cook it over medium heat, stirring constantly, until it is thick and smooth. Use a wooden spoon and be sure to stir the sauce from the bottom and sides of the pot. Let it come to a boil, then put the pot over simmering water and let it cook gently for another 10 or 15 minutes, stirring frequently. Season the sauce to taste with salt and pepper.

Wine notes
Italian: Dolcetto—Ratti
American: Merlot—Clos du Val

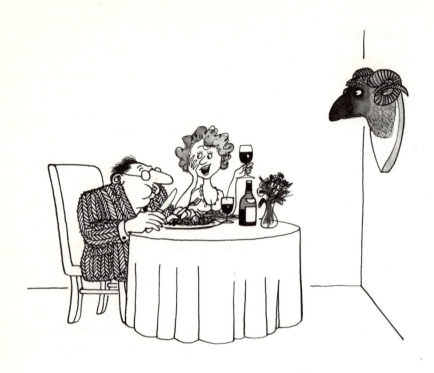

Your New Teeth

As the past recedes, memories lose some of their intensity, even those representing periods of suffering and pain. When my patients finally receive their new teeth, I often see a difference in spirit—I would almost say they look more youthful—when they come back for the first follow-up visit. The new teeth often restore a feeling of self-confidence, which may enhance mood and energy, and thus they exude a more youthful appearance. Having reached such a point not only makes the patient happy, but also the dentist, who feels professional satisfaction and pride.

What can a patient expect from freshly cemented crowns and bridges? Let us use the example of a new car: You are excited about it, but everything is very new and needs some getting used to. At first the visual element is more important than the size and power of the engine. Slowly you need to learn about and adapt to the full extent of the car's power. With the freshly cemented crowns or bridges you will notice sensitivity for a few days or even weeks. The gum can be sensitive as well, as a result of the process of cementation. The functional movements have to be practiced with the new teeth—for a little while it may feel strange to chew, and your tongue will have to adjust to working with the teeth. This period of adaptation is a given even if your dentist used all of his expertise and the dental technician reproduced exactly what the dentist asked for. Take your time eating, and follow the advice repeated throughout this book regarding the precautions that must be heeded during the first days of healing.

The major difference with implants is that they have a reduced tactile sense. You will not have the ability to sense a small piece of food on the biting surfaces because the tactile nerves between root and bone are missing. Even though a large portion of the feeling is compensated for by other structures within the oral cavity, you should be very careful at first when biting. Do not be surprised if you initially feel insecure when eating or biting. However, this loss of sensation has a silver lining, because it allows you to drink ice-cold drinks and hot beverages without worry. The sensitive tooth cervix is part of the past when you have implants.

Now you are welcome to eat and taste what you have had to stay away from for such a long time. Savor the pleasurable flavors without any of the bad dental tastes you have had to put up with, without pain when biting, without loose provisional restorations, without a shortened set of teeth, and without the obstruction of the palate—You are free!

Celebrate this happy occasion, but listen to the recommendation of your dentist regarding what is important for the longevity of your teeth.

Ossobuco alla Cipriani

Braised Veal Shanks Cipriani

Ossobuco—one of Italy's most delicious dishes—is made with shanks of milk-fed veal that are sliced and braised in a well-flavored broth until they are tender enough to eat with a fork. The name means "bone with a hole." Each slice of veal shows a cross section of the shank: a ring of meat surrounds a round section of shank bone with its center "hole" filled with marrow. After long cooking, this marrow develops its characteristic unctuous texture and incomparable flavor.

Ossobuco is traditionally served with risotto alla milanese, made with saffron. Gremolada—a garnish of chopped herbs and other seasonings—is sprinkled over the ossobuco before serving.

Ossobuco has only one drawback; it cannot be reheated the next day.

Hind shanks should be used, because they are more tender than the front ones. Have the shanks cut into 1½- to 2-inch pieces if they are whole. Leave the membrane around the shanks, it will help them keep their shape during cooking. Make a broth with meat bones and trimmings and keep it hot to use in both the ossobuco and the risotto. For added richness in the risotto, scoop the marrow out of the end pieces of the veal shanks after they are cooked. Melt this with the butter before adding the rice.

Serves 6 as a main course
½ cup olive oil or more as needed
2 veal shanks, cut into 1½- to 2-inch slices
salt
freshly ground pepper
flour for dredging
3 celery ribs, finely chopped
2 small carrots, trimmed and finely chopped
1 large onion, finely chopped
¼ pound shiitake mushrooms, finely chopped
½ cup dry white wine
1½ cups canned crushed tomatoes
2 to 4 cups hot chicken or beef stock

For the gremolada:
1 teaspoon finely chopped lemon zest
1 small garlic clove, minced
2 tablespoons chopped flat-leaf parsley
2 tablespoons chopped fresh basil
1 teaspoon chopped fresh rosemary

Heat ¼ cup of the olive oil over medium heat in a heavy flameproof casserole or Dutch oven large enough to hold the veal slices in a single layer. (Or use 2 small casseroles and heat 3 tablespoons of oil in each.) Season the veal with salt and pepper and coat the pieces with flour, shaking off any excess. When the oil is hot, add the veal pieces and cook over medium heat, turning once, until *they are browned—10 to 15 minutes. Remove the veal from the pan and set aside. Pour off the fat from the pan, wipe it with paper towels, and add 3 tablespoons of olive oil. Heat the oil over medium-high heat and add the celery, carrots, onion, and mushrooms. Cook the vegetables, stirring frequently, until they are soft—about 15 minutes. Turn up the heat, add the wine, and boil, stirring constantly, until the wine has evaporated. Stir in the crushed tomatoes and 2 cups of the hot stock. Carefully arrange the veal slices in the casserole and spoon some of the vegetable mixture over them. If the liquid does not cover the meat, add more stock. If you need more than 4 cups of stock to cover the meat, your pan is too big and you should transfer everything to a smaller casserole.*

When the liquid comes to a boil, lower the heat, cover the casserole tightly, and simmer gently for 2 to 2½ hours or until the meat is very tender when pierced with a fork. Uncover the casserole during the last 30 minutes of cooking to reduce the sauce a bit.

While the meat is cooking, chop the ingredients for the gremolada and combine them.

Ten minutes before serving, remove the meat to a deep serving platter and keep it warm. Stir in the gremolada and simmer for a minute or 2. Then spoon the sauce over the meat. Serve with risotto alla milanese (page 87).

Wine notes
Italian: Barolo—Pio Cesare
American: Merlot—Braren Pauli

Dessert

Refer to the Harry's Bar Cookbook or visit one of Arrigo Cipriani's extraordinary restaurants to experience Meringata al Limone, a scrumptious lemon meringue pie that so many have come to enjoy.

Closing Remarks

If we were able to encourage you not to deprive yourself of good food during your time of recuperation, then this book has fulfilled its purpose.

The authors wish you a successful, comfortable treatment with lifelong results.

Also, have a healthy appetite and enjoy your meals!

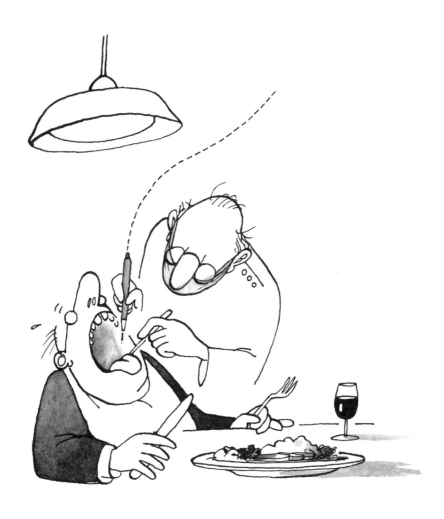

Norbert Salenbauch / Arrigo Cipriani / Volker Kriegel

Al dente

Culinary Delight for the Dental Patient
Recipes, Tips, and Advice

31.01.2012

Es lebe die Professionalität + Fun

für Feri

Norbert S.